Aging, Health,

and the

Athletic Mind Attitude

A game plan for aging and health challenges

Monty Cartwright

TABLE OF CONTENTS

PREFACE

Taking a morning shower several years ago, I noticed swollen lymph nodes in my neck that were solid and painless. This seemingly innocuous event launched a journey of twists and turns, potholes and speed bumps. At age 58, I was diagnosed with mantle cell lymphoma, an aggressive and fast-spreading cancer of the lymph system. Because of this chance early detection, my lymphoma was confined to my neck, throat, and mouth.

Once I got beyond my shock, anger, and denial, I accepted the fact that this challenge was for all the marbles. I made a conscious decision to seek inner harmony and calmness on this perilous adventure and to confront my cancer opponent with the mindset of a disciplined athlete. During my forty-year career as an athletic coach and health educator, I had discovered that how one faces a challenge is an individual decision. Others can offer advice, but ultimately it's a personal choice to adopt the attitude of an athlete-warrior or a spectator-victim. My game plan became to implement an athletic mind attitude (AMA) of effort, tenacity, and self-discipline.

Just as I had prepared physically and mentally for athletic competition, I became a patient-athlete training for survival. I went through radiation, chemotherapy, and surgery. I was in remission for almost five years before experiencing a recurrence, followed by a stem-cell transplant. In June 2006, four years after my diagnosis, I entered the San Francisco Marathon as a 62nd birthday present to myself. In the summer of 2008 I started competing in masters track and field, throwing the javelin and doing the triple jump. I went skydiving in May 2009 for my 65th birthday.

The AMA approach to getting older and living with a health challenge has worked for me and numerous others. I decided to write this book to share the AMA philosophy. It may not be for everyone, but it is my hope that it is a viable option for you. The athletic mind attitude is a proactive mental and physical approach to dealing with adversity, illness, and aging.

Too often health, aging, and wellness guidelines are presented as complex issues. The purpose of this booklet is to act as a simple, concise, and common-sense resource. In it I outline what the athletic mind attitude is, how to develop it, and how to apply it as a game plan in your life. I share advice from senior athletes I surveyed, as well as my own observations and experiences. At the back you'll find AMA terminology definitions and a resource guide with online health and aging information links.

Ultimately, this is a book about choice. Whether you have a sports participation background or not, adopting an AMA mind-set is a personal choice between being an active player or a passive fan.

Since the cancer diagnosis and as I have grown older, my life has changed. Lifestyle adjustments have been necessary. I have less energy and require periodic naps throughout the day. Dental problems, medication side-effects, and sight and hearing deterioration are a few of the trade-offs for survival.

I have also become more aware and appreciative of family, the environment, and life in the moment. In many ways I feel like a kid again and am not hesitant to seek out new adventures and experiences. I feel my life coming full circle. I realize that most of life is "bug spit" and that lost moments cannot be recaptured.

Procrastination is no longer acceptable to me. We've all had the experience of saying, "Someday I'm going to . . ." Today is my someday.

THE ATHLETIC MIND ATTITUDE (AMA)

"Keep a balance within your athleticism and your daily life. Stay focused on all positive aspects of your life. Eat and rest well."
65-year-old female, Colorado

A common definition of *athlete* is someone trained to compete in sport. An athlete possesses physical strength, agility, and endurance. Attributes such as skill, speed, balance, coordination, and technique are often also included when defining an athlete. Just as some people are gifted in art, math, or music, so are some individuals gifted in physical skill. Physical stature or hereditary traits can often predispose a person to participate in certain sports. For example, prowess in basketball is greater if one is seven feet tall. But just as being able to draw does not make one an artist nor does an innate aptitude for math qualify one as an engineer, physical ability alone does not make one an athlete.

An athlete is someone who is dedicated to the physical, mental, and intellectual rigors of training for team or individual competition. An athlete possesses an internal fortitude that transcends outcome alone. For an athlete, the process is just as important as the outcome. *Effort* is the core characteristic of an athletic personality. The emphasis is on trying and not giving up, regardless of the odds of success or failure. It is this attitude of "giving it your all" that is the foundation of the athletic mind attitude (AMA).

Possessing the attitude of an athlete is not a once-in-a-while thing but rather a consistent, proactive way of life. Positive daily habits and healthy decisions are vital components of this attitude. For older adults and individuals confronting health challenges, adoption of an athletic mind attitude can provide encouraging outcomes such as increased self-worth, confidence, better physical and mental health, and a zest for living. In addition, anxiety, doubt, and depression generally decrease with its implementation.

The athletic mind attitude is a philosophical outlook that adapts competitive sport principles, routines, and visualization techniques to day-to-day behaviors. It is exemplified by optimism, tenacity, self-determination, confidence, persistence, adaptability, composure, and adherence to ethical standards. To adopt an athletic mind attitude is to think like an athlete.

In athletics, there are many ways to achieve performance objectives. For example, some distance runners train exclusively on a program of high mileage (long-slow-distance/LSD), while others do short high-intensity intervals. Still others may incorporate a combination of both. What works best for one person may not work for somebody else, yet all can achieve success. Seasoned athletes understand themselves and do what works. The same can be said for adopting the principles of the athletic mind attitude. The key is to find which elements of the AMA approach work for you and then to incorporate them into your own life in a way that fits, making adjustments as necessary as time goes by.

Confronting the aging process and health challenges with the mind-set of a competitive athlete is a proactive coping method. The following sections provide strategies and examples of how you might apply the athletic mind attitude to aging and health challenges. (Although aging and health challenges are presented here as separate categories, the AMA strategies are transferable from one category to the other.) How you use these strategies will depend upon your individual needs and goals.

AMA STRATEGIES FOR AGING

"I have senior friends who have pacemakers, who have been through chemotherapy, have lower back problems, even bad knees, who continue to play tournament softball. They are not going to quit! They are not going to give in without a fight."
71-year-old male, Oregon

Signs of aging usually develop gradually, are diverse in nature, and fluctuate from person to person. These can include changes in skin, hair, vision, eating, hearing, balance, muscle strength, sleeping patterns, memory, libido, and urinary and bowel habits. The following AMA approaches to these changes can be a constructive way to cope and to promote healthy aging.

MAKE ANTICIPATORY DECISIONS.

Athletic intelligence includes the ability to anticipate situations and to respond appropriately in the moment without even having to think about it. *Anticipatory decisions* are decisions made beforehand in a variety of sport situations. For example, assuming the correct rebounding position in basketball is initially a conscious decision for a novice but with repetitive practice becomes a subconscious part of the game. As another example, notice how experienced football coaches have made decisions ahead of time about different situations that might occur in a game, including substitution decisions, game strategy (passing vs. running plays), and decisions about scoring attempts (touchdown vs. field goal). Emotional, spur-of-the-moment decisions are rare among seasoned coaches.

For older adults, making anticipatory decisions about lifestyle behaviors can be a major factor in successful aging. When you make a decision about healthy choices you're going to implement in advance of a situation, you end up with a feeling of self-control. For example, you can decide beforehand that you're going to walk up stairs instead of ride the elevator whenever the opportunity presents itself, or that you're going to select a snack of fruit instead of a donut, or set a limit on alcohol consumption. When you adhere to them consistently over time, such simple choices add up to a comprehensive wellness profile. Just as correct rebounding position eventually becomes automatic for a basketball player, so can predetermined lifestyle choices become automatic for the older adult with an athletic mind attitude.

GIVE YOUR DAILY WELLNESS ROUTINES PRIORITY STATUS.

Usually, at some point in an athletic career, athletes must decide how important their sport is to them. Are the sacrifices required really worth it? There is no right or wrong answer, but the decision to commit 100 percent to a sport and to make it a priority distinguishes an athlete from a recreational player. Athletes know that to reach their performance potential, they must reduce or totally eliminate negative and distracting behaviors. Making healthy choices and being aware of priorities is a cornerstone of the athletic personality. Self-esteem, an optimistic demeanor, and self-confidence are accompanying attributes.

Healthy aging requires the same approach. Giving priority to exercise, diet, and sleep is an important decision for a senior citizen. The aging body is not as forgiving of negative habits as the youthful body. Just as you wouldn't voluntarily skip meals or deprive yourself of sleep each day, you should not assign daily wellness routines secondary status.

KNOW YOUR LIMITS.

The livelihood of a professional tennis player depends on performing at a maximum level in numerous tournaments. Seldom will professional players place themselves in a situation that jeopardizes their career, such as diving head-first for a ball, leaping into the stands during a volley, or letting competitive intensity get out of control. They have mentally conditioned themselves to do their best within skill and safety boundaries. Most athletes know their limits. Rarely will they "push the envelope" to the point of risking a career-ending injury.

Applying the same approach is beneficial for older adults. Tempering habits and activities that you once took for granted (like sun tanning and climbing ladders) becomes important. The mental mind-set of not overdoing a good thing in order to do it again and again prevails among senior athletes. Enjoyment and safety are enhanced through self-control and restraint. A simple guideline to follow is: whenever in doubt, do less.

USE THE FIT FORMULA.

For senior athletes, determining the minimal frequency, intensity, and time (duration) necessary to make an exercise pay off is important. This is known as the FIT formula. The objective of FIT is to incorporate the components of fitness—cardio-respiratory endurance, muscular strength, and flexibility—into a structured weekly routine.

- **Frequency** refers to how many times a week you will exercise. For the beginner, the minimum frequency is three times per week.

- **Intensity** is the effort factor. When starting out, go easy. For example, walk instead of run. Using your heart rate as a guide to intensity of effort is a good way to monitor a workout session. Follow this formula: 220 minus your age equals the maximum exercise heart rate (MHR) in beats per minute (bpm). Avoid working beyond this MHR and instead stay within your exercise heart rate (EHR) range, which is between 50 percent (beginner) and 80 percent (advanced) of the MHR. For example, for a fit 70 year old the MHR is 220–70=150 bpm and the EHR is 150 × 80% = 120 bpm.

- **Time** (duration) is how long an exercise session lasts. Most trainers recommend a minimum of thirty minutes of activity for endurance and strength-building exercises such as weight training and Pilates.

As a starting point for FIT, establish a personal baseline that follows general physical fitness principles. For the sedentary older person just beginning an exercise program, a medical exam and consultation with a certified trainer is recommended. For the competitive athlete, the FIT formula is adjusted according to training cycle objectives. Choosing activities that you enjoy and that meet your special needs will help you adhere to your activity program.

Remember that physical fitness training formulas such as FIT should serve as general guidelines and are not absolute. A recommended approach to intensity for all types of exercise is to go by *perceived exertion*—that is, awareness of how you feel. Also, it is important to include rest as part of the workout program.

USE PROPER TECHNIQUE.

An athlete knows the importance of correct body mechanics in a successful performance. Applying the proper technique leads to proficiency. Observe an accomplished figure skater, golfer, or wrestler and note their ease of movement and skill execution. This excellence occurs because they incorporate correct biomechanics.

Proper sport technique rarely changes. Occasionally, refinement and corrections may have to be made. Accomplished athletes achieve this through consultation and use of reminders that may include mental visualization rituals, written reminders, and/

or verbalizing key words. Listening to an audiotape through headphones is another proven method to remind an athlete of proper body mechanics.

These same principles can apply to older individuals. For example, when you walk, observe your posture and whether your body is in alignment. Are you moving with ease or are you off balance or shuffling? Where are you looking? What is the position of your head? Just as an athlete uses reminders, you can use technique cues. For example, if you say to yourself, "Chin up" or "Look straight ahead" as you walk, you will find that your body assumes a more erect posture. Your shoulders are less slumped and your hips correctly lead your body forward. By swinging your arms with each step, you will automatically extend your stride and eliminate shuffling.

REMEMBER THESE SIMPLE REMINDERS ABOUT AGING AND HEALTH.

- The three pillars of health are exercise, diet, and sleep.

- Food + exercise + genetics = your body. (Hope Heart Institute)

- Set goals that are specific and can be measured.

- Aim for seventy minutes of activity per week to reduce your risk of major disease and improve your quality of life. The psychological benefits can be as profound as the physical benefits. (Pennington Research Center)

- Remember that intensity of exercise is a key factor in weight control. Walking thirty minutes at 4 mph on a flat surface will burn 135 calories; walking up a hill will burn 200 calories.

- The single best way to prevent illness is to wash your hands both before and after almost any activity—eating, sex, toileting, sneezing/coughing, gardening, wound care, animal petting, diaper changing, touching (door handles, handshakes, and so forth). Avoid or minimize face touching. (University of California Wellness Newsletter)

- Get annual flu shots, tetanus boosters every ten years, and hepatitis A shots if you travel. Vaccines you received when you were younger may wear off and leave you more susceptible to infections like pneumonia or the flu. (Comprehensive Blood and Cancer Center)

- To help with memory, keep lists, limit multitasking, and think in groups (items/categories/numbers). Automatically put essential items like keys and glasses in the same place every time. (UCLA Center on Aging)

- Once you replace negative thoughts with positive ones, you'll start having positive re-sults. (Willie Nelson)

- A great prescription for life: laugh, love, and live in the moment.

AMA STRATEGIES FOR HEALTH CHALLENGES

"It is very important to have a good attitude and stay healthy. Eat healthy foods, don't drink or smoke. Have a positive attitude in all things."
87-year-old female, Oregon

Thinking like an athlete can play an important part in dealing with health challenges. An athlete is engaged, not passive. A patient-athlete cultivates a mental attitude that incorporates hope, resiliency, adaptability, and calmness. I used the following AMA strategies during my journey to survive cancer.

KNOW YOUR OPPONENT.

A coach will study and scout the opponent. Understanding the strengths and weaknesses of the competition is a valuable asset. Knowledge enhances game preparation and planning. The same principle applies to confronting a disease or illness. The vast amount of information available on the Internet can serve as a base for inquiry and discussion with medical professionals. Look up your condition and learn as much as you can about it.

At the same time, watch out for faulty information or outright quackery. Do not accept things blindly. Maintain a healthy suspicion. If it seems too good to be true, be wary. Confirm research information with sources you believe and trust such as your family doctor or other credible health professional. My wife, a PhD nurse educator, was my screening expert for questionable data.

SEEK ADVICE.

Consulting with people who have had similar challenges can be immensely helpful, especially during the treatment phase of a disease. Gaining an understanding of how other people have competed against a common opponent will lessen your fear of the unknown. Like a game-changing pep talk, their experience can inspire your courage. You can find support groups and/or individuals through government health offices, Internet searches, and local medical centers, and by putting the word out through family and friends. I was able to make contact with supportive people through the American Cancer Society, lymphoma support organizations, and local cancer affiliates.

BE PREPARED FOR SURPRISES.

No matter how much an athlete prepares for an opponent, the unexpected can occur. Competitive athletes adjust with resiliency and flexibility. Incorporating an athletic mind attitude allows the patient-athlete to navigate unexpected diagnostic and treatment surprises with minimal anxiety. Both an athlete and a patient-athlete know that unforeseen circumstances are the norm. A baseball hitter may anticipate a fastball only to be thrown a curve. Good hitters adjust. When blood clots appeared during my chemo treatments, new medications were prescribed to correct the problem. Mentally adjusting to bruising and bleeding was challenging but doable. An attitude of expecting the unexpected is a positive way for the patient-athlete to move forward.

TRAIN PHYSICALLY AND MENTALLY.

Physical and mental training are dependent upon each other. To fully achieve one's athletic potential, a person must practice each. To successfully confront health issues, the patient-warrior incorporates both each day into healing rituals.

Physical fitness has four components: cardiovascular, joint flexibility, muscle strength, and muscle endurance. You can train in each of these components during and after treatment for illness. Of course, you will need to adjust the intensity and frequency of your exercise as your health circumstances fluctuate. Consistency is the key factor in maintaining physical fitness. Realistically, what counts is not the specific exercises you do but rather the effort of doing something each and every day. For example, when first diagnosed I could bench press 200 lbs. During treatment, as I became more frail, I attempted to maintain my bench press routine by lying in bed and moving my arms without any weights. Mentally, I envisioned I was pushing 200 lbs. Today I can bench press 125 lbs.

An athlete knows that the mental component of training and competition is just as essential as the physical in achieving performance goals. A positive mental attitude—incorporating self-discipline, tenacity, focus, and dedication—is the key to unlocking physical potential. A negative mental approach—excuses, blame, self-doubt, quitting, and so on—creates downbeat results. Often, a positive mind-set begins with confident, upbeat word usage. Words can inspire action and mental toughness.

Many athletes and coaches use personal mantras and aphorisms as the catalyst for an upbeat attitude. Word choice may vary from person to person but all tend to have the following common characteristics: they are brief, they are personal, and they inspire. Each day I remind myself that I am a warrior-athlete (which suggests that I have the tenacity and determination of a fighter, that I am not passive or submissive, and that I do not give up), repeat the phrase "good health flows from inner calm," and read inspirational comments. Uplifting music and affirmative visualization routines can also empower a positive attitude. Negative mental stress, on the other hand, can adversely impact athletic performance and hamper survival chances. Stress siphons curative forces from the healing process. Remove these hurdles and the physical race becomes more manageable.

ASSEMBLE A MEDICAL TEAM.

An athlete has a better chance of success when taught by a special-event coach (whether that event is pitching, pole vaulting, or something else). The same principle applies to the patient-athlete when working with a medical team. Choose medical personnel and hospitals equipped to give the best care for your specific medical ailment.

During my initial diagnosis phase, I spent considerable time talking with a variety of medical specialists. I sought out people who provided the expertise and compatibility that would enhance my survival chances. Once I had my team in place, I might occasionally question some procedure, but generally I entrusted myself to their care, just as an athlete would with a respected and trusted coach. I tried to follow this same principle with nurses, technicians, and auxiliary personnel. If I did not feel comfortable or confident with my medical team, I sought change.

ENLIST TEAMMATE SUPPORT.

Fostering positive relationships with family and friends enhances healing. In both sports and healing, success depends on the performance of the whole squad, not just the star player. Team members include spouses, children, friends, counselors, spiritual advisors, work colleagues, dieticians, and the like. Communication with team members is essential. When the team knows the guidelines for care and support of the patient-athlete, good things are possible. Sometimes well-intended gestures by support teammates may hinder healing. For example, because of my compromised immune system, I had to avoid handshakes, hugs, crowds, and homemade foods. My teammates understood and respected these guidelines.

Support from teammates can enhance healing for the patient-athlete. Let others know you need them. For me, simple gifts, music CDs, sharing of funny movie titles, and occasional silly cards had magical healing power. Receiving a phone call or e-mail message from someone who just wanted to say hello did wonders for my mental outlook. Teammates can assure you that you have not been forgotten. Teammates can also understand and help you deal with the downsides that accompany health issues. For example, during the hard times when I suffered mental depression and physical setbacks, my wife never wavered in her support. Her mere presence in good and bad times, spoken words of encouragement, touches, and gestures of love and kindness guided me through some rough times. Caregivers can be the forgotten cohort along the patient-athlete's journey to recovery.

BE AN ACTIVE PARTICIPANT.

Know and try to understand what is happening to you. The best healer is one's self, comparable to the captain of a team. You will suffer much less emotional anxiety during and after treatment if you are involved in decisions and planning.

BE AWARE OF TREATMENT CONSEQUENCES.

In a sporting contest, knowledge beforehand can make a challenging situation tolerable. This information helps an athlete prepare mentally for rough workouts and the game ahead. This also applies to the patient-athlete. Unpleasant treatment can become more bearable when you know what outcomes to expect. For me, chemotherapy and radiation were bearable because I knew a positive outcome was possible.

MAKE AN EFFORT AND HAVE PATIENCE.

In athletics, effort is the primary catalyst for success. Athletes do not compete halfheartedly every once in awhile. They do their best every time. This effort mind-set is an essential part of AMA. For some it may be making an effort to walk ten steps farther than a week ago or simply turning in bed without assistance. For others it may be preparing for an extended bike trip, competing in senior sports competitions, or fighting the urge to become a couch potato. Active physical and mental engagement plays a prominent role in the healing process.

In addition, an athlete knows that worthy athletic endeavors cannot be accomplished in haste.

Patience is an unspoken virtue. A deliberate, calm, and tenacious approach to skill and technique development improves the odds of performance success. This is a vital mind-set adopted by AMA participants.

ALLOW TIME FOR RECOVERY AND HEALING.

After a grueling marathon, tennis tournament, or long sports season, an athlete will rest and recuperate before returning to competition. Doing too much too soon rarely accomplishes anything in the short or long term. The same is true for the patient-athlete. Active rest—consciously rebuilding the body and mind through limited physical exertion, nutritious food, adequate hydration, and sufficient sleep—can be a prescription for survival.

SET AN EXAMPLE.

Cancer survivor and Tour de France champion Lance Armstrong has said, "An athlete has to figure how to enrich others; otherwise he is purposeless." Dedicated athletes know that actions speak louder than words. The patient-athlete can be a role model who demonstrates how to face adversity.

Demonstrating courage and dignity sets a positive example for others as they face their own challenges and struggles.

BE YOUR OWN COACH

"Develop a weekly routine that you enjoy, then stay with it."
59-year-old male, Indiana

During the early stages of an athlete's career, the coach plays a significant role in setting guidelines for physical conditioning, skill development, and sport strategy. This mentor-student relationship is generally a positive chapter in an athlete's development. The coach's experience, training, and knowledge greatly influence future potential growth of the young athlete. Although often dictatorial in nature, this stage can establish a constructive foundation for future growth.

With maturity, the athlete develops into an autonomous learner, the coach becomes a consultant, and sports participation reflects goals influenced by career and social criteria. The vast majority of senior athletes spend very little, if any, time with a coach-mentor. Whether by circumstances or default, most older athletes become

their own coaches as they age. The same principle may apply to non-athletes: as we age, lifestyle
decisions and actions are more and more up to
us. Each of us ultimately determines how we will
approach this stage of life.

For older self-coached athletes, training physically can be relatively simple. Select a favorite sport,
evaluate personal goals and capabilities, draw
upon past experience, and seek advice from others.
This model can also be adopted by older adults for
wellness goals. Just as an athlete adjusts as needed
when training for competition, so should a senior be
flexible and resilient during this stage of life.

For both the athlete and the older person, there
is always an excuse to not do something. The AMA
solution to such a dilemma is not to give up but to
find a way to make things work or explore alter-
native ways to achieve goals. For example, severe
knee joint problems may limit a runner. Substituting
deep water pool running or treadmill intervals with
limited flat surface grass runs may prolong this athlete's running career. If not, adopting another type
of activity may be necessary to achieve fitness and
competitive goals.

Sport skill and technique development generally follows planned systematic practice routines.
An athlete incorporates the same sequential principles of physical conditioning into mental attitude

development. An ultra distance runner gradually increases mileage and calluses as he molds his mind and body to the demands of this grueling endurance sport. An Olympic weight lifting competitor prepares for each incremental poundage increase mentally before performing it physically. Older adults can apply the same approach to wellness goals—incorporating lifestyle changes in a planned incremental manner.

You can imitate this athletic mind-body approach to train your attitude by setting and working toward goals and objectives over a period of time. Positive affirmations, associating with upbeat people, and being mindful to live in the moment are essential ingredients in the attitude development process. Attitude training also includes eliminating negative words and negative thinking and replacing them with more optimistic words and thoughts. This may be easier said than done, but you will never know if you can change your mental habits unless you try. Do something often enough and it eventually becomes a habit. Attitude development is a deliberate, conscious process. For the senior citizen it requires the same dedication and time commitment as it requires of a champion marathoner.

For the self-coached person, it is imperative to follow established mind-body improvement principles. The following are building blocks to incorporate into a self-coaching model. They include a two-pronged approach: knowledge acquisition and common sense application.

COMMON WELLNESS GUIDELINES

- Use the FIT—frequency, intensity, time (duration)—formula for fitness training. In order to attain fitness, you must exercise often, with effort, and for a duration that will reap physiological benefits.

- Know your BMR—basal metabolic rate. This calculation serves as a calorie expenditure guide based on your activity level.

- Use your heart rate—resting, exercise, recovery—as a personal fitness monitor. Knowing your resting heart rate (beats per minute for 60 seconds), exercise heart rate (level of recommended exertion), and recovery rate (how quickly your heartbeat count decreases) gives you an objective method of evaluation.

WELLNESS CONSISTENCY

- Establish daily wellness (mind, body, spirit) routines. Consistency of effort is the single most important factor in achieving athletic and wellness success. Doing something each day toward your goals, no matter how small, will garner rewards.

- Make wellness a priority in your life. Ask yourself: How important is [fill in the blank] to me, on a scale of one to ten? A designation of eight and above indicates priority status for you. Act accordingly.

- Create healthy habits—add positive and subtract negative behaviors. The more you incorporate positive behaviors, the more these actions become part of your personality. The same can be said for negative behaviors.

PHYSICAL FITNESS AND SPORT TRAINING

- Identify the whole and work on the parts. In other words, to achieve athletic skill, work on specific aspects that make up the skill. For example, a golf swing is composed of multiple techniques (stance, head position, back swing, and so forth). Improvement of a golf swing occurs when each of these technical parts is mastered and put together as a whole.

- Remember that every workout has both specific and general goals. During a weight lifting session, for instance, a specific goal would be to do a certain number of bench presses. The general goal would be to strengthen your chest muscles.

- Doing less more often is better than more less often. The body and mind will adjust to gradual, but consistent, stimulus. The body recovers more quickly and generally performs at a higher level of efficiency when workouts are concise with an emphasis on quality. The opposite occurs when practices are longer in duration and/or done less frequently. For example, trying to make up missed short workouts in fewer training sessions of longer duration creates a formula for injury, frustration, and quitting. And it isn't fun!

BODY MECHANICS

- Understand the biomechanics of your selected activities and follow proper body mechanics. A basic understanding of how your muscular and skeletal systems work is invaluable. Correct application of biomechanical principles aids athletic performance. For example, in throwing the discus, an extended lever (arm) enhances flight distance.

- Do not sacrifice proper technique for immediate results. Improper technique stymies improvement as well as inviting injury. Poor habits are hard to break. A golf swing is more that just the ability to hit a stationary ball—it is a complex athletic skill. If the skill is sacrificed to merely hit the ball for distance, future improvement is jeopardized. Practicing poor technique insures that the golfer will become very good at being a bad duffer.

- Learn to move, move to learn. There is a positive correlation between body awareness and mental acuteness. How one moves (running, throwing, skipping, and so on) influences cognitive functioning. Learning correct body position and movement principles creates a positive learning and activity environment.

INJURIES

- There is no such thing as a minor injury. Injuries for an athlete are a given. The key is to limit the degree of the injury. It is wiser to err on the side of caution in regard to injuries. Treat all injuries as potentially serious.

- Practice RICE—rest, ice, compress, elevate. A few minutes of immediate care decreases recovery time.

- Accept that recovery is incremental and gradual. Healing is a process. Very few things, including injury recovery, are achieved in haste.

NUTRITION

- Eat to live, don't live to eat. Avoid eating for entertainment.

- Read food labels—know what you consume. Improvement in eating habits is not possible without baseline knowledge of what you are consuming.

- Limit your intake of sugar, salt, saturated fat, and fried foods.

STRESS MANAGEMENT

- Identify stressors—people and/or situations. Avoid negative influences whenever possible; if not possible, minimize exposure.

- Implement personal stress-reduction activities. Know yourself. Identify healthy activities and do them whenever stress becomes overwhelming.

- Seek balance in all things—diet, relationships, rest, exercise, and so on. Feeling off kilter can often be traced to overindulgence. More does not mean better. Seek quality over quantity.

EMOTIONAL HEALTH

- Humor is a powerful anti-aging medicine. Laugh often and loud or a least giggle and smile in silence.

- Adequate sleep and rest enhances emotional stability. Regardless of an athlete's skill proficiency, he or she cannot perform effectively without adequate rest. Rest fills the energy tank. Without it, the fuel tank will run dry.

- Live in the moment and take pleasure in the five senses: hearing, seeing, touching, tasting, smelling. Awareness of self and surroundings is a key that unlocks potential.

THINK LIKE AN ATHLETE: YOUR AMA PLAYBOOK

"Set realistic goals and keep revising them."
80-year-old male

Very few noteworthy things in sports happen by chance. Preparation is the key to successful athletic performance, as well as success in other fields, whether it be business, medicine, or politics. The individual who possesses vision, organization, and self-discipline will be successful. This same principle applies to aging and meeting health challenges. Just as running a marathon requires a systematic and incremental approach to training, so too does implementation of the athletic mind attitude and positive aging practices.

To outline your own personal approach to achieving your goals in an organized and systematic way, I suggest that you create an AMA playbook. This is where you record your game plan. You are much more likely to achieve goals that you have written down, so a playbook gives you a place to write down your goals and track your progress. The playbook will help you solidify and strengthen behaviors you wish to incorporate in your life. It is a valuable tool that will provide guidance, keep your program on target, and give you reference benchmarks. It will enhance your efforts as you develop an athletic personality.

No two people are alike; no two people have the same goals or methods of attainment. The same can be said about creation and use of an AMA playbook. Just as seasoned coaches adapt basic principles, proven teaching guidelines, and dependable strategies to fit their individual coaching philosophy, you will customize your own AMA playbook.

Here's how to create your own custom AMA playbook.

1. Identify lifestyle goals or current habits you want to maintain or improve.

You may first need to gather basic information about the primary areas of wellness—mind, body, and spirit—to identify changes you want to make and new goals you want to establish. For example, your goals may be in the area of exercise, stress reduction, or nutrition. Make your goals specific and measurable.

2. Decide how you can best accomplish your goal(s).

Outline schedules and routines you will follow. Make anticipatory decisions. For example, if you want to live more aerobically, this may mean establishing internal mental reminders to take the stairs instead of the elevator or bike to work instead of driving. Or you may choose to outline your game plan through charting, checklists, or journaling. Observe athletic competitors and coaches and notice how some use clipboards, wrist notations, or audio recordings. Written technique reminders on 5×7 cards are also helpful. Do what works.

3. Consciously implement behavior changes.

This requires self-discipline and the conviction that the identified goals are very important. In this phase of the game plan, simple and regular actions are essential. The goal is to create positive habits. For example, if your goal is nutrition improvement, your new habits may include drinking fat-free milk, limiting salt intake, and avoiding fried food whenever possible. Exceptions to the playbook objectives should be rare.

4. Edit the playbook as needed.

It's best to keep the playbook simple and to make it personal and adaptable for age and health changes.

SENIOR ATHLETE AMA SURVEY

*"Don't get suckered into the common beliefs
on aging. You can start being an athlete
at any age."*
55-year-old female

I conducted a survey of 110 older athletes over a period of five-plus years to find out why some older adults remain active and engaged while others do not. Senior athletes exemplify a "can do" attitude. I was curious to find out more about the mental attitude of this segment of the population and how they approach health and aging challenges. I hoped to confirm my belief that older athletes could be an example and an inspiration to others. My employer, Southern Oregon University in Ashland, Oregon, was supportive and provided technical assistance for the survey.

Respondents to the survey questions included both females (43 of them) and males (63 of them), ranging in age from 50 to 91 years; the average age was 63. Geographical representation was widespread: most of the respondents lived in the Pacific Northwest (25 percent), followed by the East (20 percent), the Midwest and South (16 percent), and the West (15 percent). Twenty-three percent didn't designate their geographic location, and 1 percent were from international locations.

I asked the respondents to list all sports activities in which they participated, both competitively and on a recreational basis. Multiple activities were common. The top ten ranked sports were weight training, biking, golf, swimming, basketball, tennis, road racing (running), cross-country, track and field, and triathlon, in that order. Other activities mentioned included baseball, basketball, bowling, gardening, racquetball, downhill skiing, table tennis, and yoga, among others.

I asked four open-ended questions to uncover information about the value of sports participation in the lives of the respondents. Common themes emerged regarding life attitudes and views about health, illness, and aging. The survey findings support the premise that an optimistic attitude, combined with physical activity, results in a healthier lifestyle. These findings, along with interviews and discussions I conducted with masters athletes, reinforce the importance of the mind-body connection. Attempting to improve the health of one without also including the other is like an athlete competing in swimming without ever practicing in the water.

Here are the four questions and a summary of the responses I received:

1. What advice would you give others about being a competitive senior athlete and about leading an active lifestyle?

- A personal commitment to activity and a nutritious diet reaps positive benefits. In addition to feeling better, relationships and self-esteem are enhanced.

- The quantity of years is not guaranteed, but the quality of life is.

- Being a competitive athlete is fun.

2. What is your favorite motivational saying regarding participation and competition in athletic events?

- The Nike theme "Just do it" emerged as the most common mantra. The idea is that making no excuses and engaging in competitive games far outweighs any pitfalls such as aches, pain, and soreness.

- "Ignore the nay-sayers." Strong-willed and opinionated, senior athletes realize that they are the ones in control of their personal destinies.

- "Use it or lose it" permeates a majority of responses. Being sedentary, both mentally and physically, is a detriment in this phase of life.

3. As an older athlete, how important is attitude and your mental approach to athletic competition, exercise, and physical fitness?

- One is not possible without the other.

4. How has being an athlete helped you with health challenges as you have gotten older?

- Involvement in training and competing helps take the mind off health problems. You don't mope around, complain as much, or worry as often.

- Sport activity helps improve and maintain health, and slow down health deterioration. Stated examples included weight control, osteoporosis, cancer (prevention and treatment), heart disease, and joint/muscle problems.

- "You look and feel better" was stated multiple times in the survey.

FINAL WORDS

At the end of this book I'd like to leave you with some wise words from the senior athletes who took part in this survey. Their comments offer us hope that cultivating an athletic mind attitude – thinking and acting like an athlete – can promote health, balance and happiness at all stages of life's journey.

"I started running when I was 62 years old. I have completed 227 races, winning 225 in my five-year age group, including three mini-marathons. You are never too old to get in better shape." 68-year-old male, Indiana

"Fitness and nutrition (barring disease) really are the fountain of youth. Fitness is simple, but not easy. Good things take effort." 58-year-old female, Colorado

"An active lifestyle is important, but remember that you are not 30 or 40 years old anymore so don't try to train as though you were. I don't run or ski more than three days a week. I cross-train the other two or three days (weights, yoga, etcetera). I think many master athletes over train." 91-year-old male, Oregon

"You may be slower and have some aches and pains afterward, but the aches and pains are worth being able to keep moving. Your attitude will improve, your health will improve, and your life will improve through contact with friends and the pleasure of participating. This will make life so much more enjoyable!" 61-year-old female, Iowa

"Worry less about being competitive and more about just doing something." 52-year-old male, California

"There is nothing better for you physically or mentally than to be active. And don't be prideful. You are going to slow down, but the doing is still fun." 56-year-old female, Montana

"Being physically active has increased my self-esteem and endurance. I catch fewer colds. Know your body and its limitations. It's all right to be mediocre in an activity and enjoy it. Try new things." 55-year-old female, Ohio

"Just do it and enjoy a healthier life. Gain energy, friendship, respect, and a healthy sex life." 70-year-old male

"Staying active is a requirement for maintaining a healthy mind and body. I would say the health benefits alone outweigh some of the limitations/ aches that come with aging." 60-year-old male, Illinois

"With retirement and growing older we now have the time to play and be active. Most don't and they miss out on so much." 58-year-old male, British Columbia, Canada

"Being physically active is an important part of maintaining a balanced lifestyle (the others being intellectual, emotional, and social stimulation)." 62-year-old male, New York

"Modifying activity is necessary. Don't let anyone or anything discourage you!" 65-year-old female, Connecticut

"Mix your preparation by working via treadmill and free weights as well as your sport." 65-year-old male, Georgia

"Cross-training is essential. Treat aches and muscle injuries immediately and monitor your recovery. Eat and drink well." 56-year-old female, Texas

"Try to find a training partner or group to exercise, train, or compete with. Compete for the love of the sport and the friendships that follow." 55-year-old male, Massachusetts

"Physical activity makes life worth living. It enables you to keep your weight where you want it and look younger." 83-year-old female, North Carolina

"Get up and get out." 69-year-old male, California

AMA TERMINOLOGY

Active rest: The process of recovery that involves diminished physical activity. Consciously rebuilding the body and mind through diet, rest, and meditation.

Anticipatory decision: Decision made beforehand about how to react/behave in common situations.

Athletic intelligence: Intrinsic physical and cognitive performance traits, such as balance, coordination, skill, strategies, and adaptability, that manifest themselves in both sport and everyday settings. These are often instinctive but can also be learned through experience and practice.

Athletic mind attitude (AMA): A mind-set of self-discipline that incorporates attributes of sport rituals, competition, and physical fitness. A mental method using principles and strategies from sports to help meet the challenges of illness and aging.

Athletic personality: Traits include optimism, tenacity, self-esteem, confidence, persistence, competitiveness, and adherence to ethical stand-ards. All foster the athletic mind attitude.

Negative mental stress: Aspects of one's lifestyle that are absent of redeeming virtues and that add up to have a harmful impact on emotional and physical health.

Patient-athlete: A person undergoing medical challenges who purposefully adopts the mental attitude of an athlete, including hope, resiliency, adaptability, and calmness.

Think like an athlete: To approach daily situa-tions and decisions—such as those involving diet and nutrition, exercise, and teamwork—using AMA principles.

Warrior-athlete: A person who incorporates an athletic mental attitude with the tenacity and determination of a fighter; someone who is neither passive nor submissive and does not give up.

POSITIVE AGING RESOURCES

"I may not live any longer, but my wife says I look better in my cycling outfit."
75-year-old male, Nevada

Here are some links to helpful resources on the topic of healthy aging. You can access information about specific sports competitions (such as track and field, horseshoes, or swimming) by contacting individual sports organizations. Information about specific diseases is accessible by contacting national and regional organizations (such as the American Cancer Society or the American Heart Association).

AMERICAN ASSOCIATION OF RETIRED PERSONS

www.aarp.org

An all-inclusive website for seniors that contains current information about health, finances, travel, insurance, discounts, family, online community, leisure, and current events. Includes membership sign-up.

AMERICAN COLLEGE OF SPORTS MEDICINE

www.acsm.org

Offers information and resources for the general public about federal physical activity guidelines; starting exercise programs; tips on fitness, exercise, and consumer products; information on sports medicine; and specific fitness resources and links for women, youth, and seniors.

AMERICAN SOCIETY ON AGING

www.asaging.org

Offers educational programs on aging, publications such as *Aging Today*, and information and training resources for those who work with seniors, all with the goal of improving the quality of life of older adults.

ASSOCIATION OF CANCER ONLINE RESOURCES

www.acor.org

A unique collection of online communities that provides timely and accurate information in a supportive environment. Gives access to approximately 160 mailing lists that offer support, information, and community to everyone affected by cancer and related disorders.

HELPGUIDE.ORG: HOW TO SLEEP BETTER

www.helpguide.org/life/sleep_tips.htm

Offers information on the importance of good sleep and how to get it. Covers how much sleep you need, what happens when you don't get it, as well as seven ways to improve your sleep habits.

HELPGUIDE.ORG: SENIOR NUTRITION

www.helpguide.org/life/senior_nutrition.htm

Offers healthy eating tips for older adults, including specific nutritional recommendations, dealing with loss of appetite, places for seniors to share meals, tips on changing old eating habits to improve diet, as well as a great list of related websites about senior nutrition.

MAYOCLINIC:
STRESS MANAGEMENT

**www.mayoclinic.com/health/
stress-management/MY00435/TAB=indepth**

All-encompassing page on the Mayo Clinic website that allows you to click through to other pages detailing basic information about wide-ranging techniques for stress relief including relaxation exercises. Highlights include how social support, laughter, spirituality, positive thinking, and relaxation techniques such as meditation, tai chi, and exercise can reduce stress.

NATIONAL COUNCIL ON AGING

www.ncoa.org

Provides current information for seniors on improving health, enhancing economic security, promoting independence and dignity, strengthening community, elder justice, learning opportunities, connecting with peers, community action and volunteering, home equity, long-term services and support, senior centers, chronic disease, mental health, fall prevention, and physical activity.

NATIONAL SENIOR GAMES

www.nsga.com

Includes competition in archery, badminton, bowling, cycling, golf, race walking, racquetball, road racing, softball, swimming, table tennis, track and field, triathlon, and volleyball. To compete in the National Senior Games you must be 50 years old or older and qualify by competing in state games.

NIHSENIORHEALTH

nihseniorhealth.gov/index.html

A comprehensive website offering information on healthy aging and more. Healthy aging topics include information on exercise and physical activity for older adults, sleep and aging, eating well, and helpful tips on challenges with balance, smell, and taste. The type font on this website can be increased with the click of a button, and it includes videos for easy and fun access to important information.

ACKNOWLEDGMENTS

I thank the following individuals for their help with the writing of *Aging, Health, and the Athletic Mind Attitude:*

- Dawn Thompson, Julie Cartwright, and Lorraine Anderson for their editorial assistance.

- Dyan and Cole Thompson for their technical assistance.

- Katherine Bjork for her helpful advice with the e-book version of this book.

- Southern Oregon University, Dr. Donna Mills, and Richard Rosenthal for survey support.

- The 110 senior athlete survey participants for their response and inspiration.

ABOUT THE AUTHOR

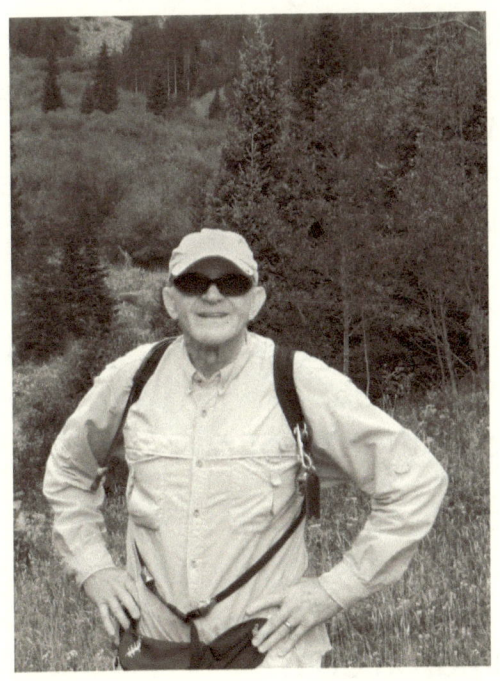

Monty Cartwright is an emeritus professor of health and physical education at Southern Oregon University in Ashland, Oregon. After thirty-plus years of living in the historic town of Jacksonville, Oregon, he and his wife, Julie, now live in Colorado Springs, Colorado, near their grandchildren.

His teaching, coaching, and athletic administrative career spans a forty-year period at the high school, community college, and university levels. He is a nationally ranked senior track athlete, a fly fisherman, and a published author. He was inducted into the Southern Oregon University Sports Hall of Fame in 2010.

His writings have appeared in *Oregon Healthy Living* magazine, *Oregon Stories Anthology*, and *Thresholds Literary Journal*. His semi-annual poetry and photography website can be viewed at www. WritingsbyMonty.com. For additional information about the AMA approach to life, access his AMA blog at Athleticmindattitude.blogspot.com.

Monty Cartwright is available for workshops and lectures about the Athletic Mind Attitude. For information send an e-mail directly to Monty at: athleticmindattitude@hotmail.com

Additional copies of this book and an e-book version are available at: www.create space.com/3570779, www.WritingsbyMonty.com and www.amazon.com.